IN TOUCH WITH
Reiki I

IN TOUCH WITH
Reiki I

A Manual for Teachers and Students

Usui Reiki I

~

Susan Rea Caldwell
Master/Teacher

Copyright © 2007
by Susan Rea Caldwell

4creatingpaths@gmail.com

All rights reserved

ISBN: 978-1-5374882-3-3

No part of this book may be reproduced in any form or by any electronic or mechanical means, including information storage and retrieval systems, without written permission from the author, except for the use of brief quotations in a book review.

Anything and everything stated in this workbook is from the experience of Susan Rea Caldwell. It is meant to give you, the reader, the student of Reiki, guidelines. Accept and reject at your own discretion. Follow your own truth, your path.

The information in this book references healing which is a different discipline than medicine. In no way do I offer medical advice or wish to discredit the medical community. In case of serious illness *always* consult your physician. Inform your physician of your use of Reiki in your health care program.

~ Dedication ~

This book is dedicated to all my Reiki teachers. Especially, Jim Adams and Antoinette Zachem, my Reiki Master. As I learned and as we received our attunements, the role of student and teacher spiraled and changed many times, as it often will.

This book would not be possible without the dedication of many to this project and to my pathwork.

Much heartfelt thanks to my revision editor, Julie Buchanan. Her suggestions blessed my project. Many times, the blessings were tough to uncover through the revisions and soul searching while plodding the thousands of steps it takes to complete a manuscript.

Finally, I would like to thank my Reiki Guides and the Angels who worked with me to process this text to publication, and those who assist me while I am sending Reiki. Their dedication and availability are vital. I honor your journey and I am certainly honored to be a part of it. Namaste.

**May all good come to you.
Peace to you and yours.
Bless you, the reader, and the connection
we now have through Reiki.**

~
**Above all else
be true to your source and yourself.**

Any student of Reiki considering working on other people should check their local requirements about touching
another person's body.

I am a licensed minister through the Universal Brotherhood. Being a minister allows me permission in the state of Kentucky. I also am insured to protect myself and any establishment where I have a Reiki studio.

~ Contents ~

1. Blessing the monetary exchange 13
2. Welcome to Reiki 15
3. New Reiki information 23
4. How Reiki works 27
5. The history of Reiki 33
6. What makes Reiki different
    from other healing modalities? 43
7. The Raku 45
8. The Reiki principles 47
9. The process of the first attunement 49
10. The first attunement 53
11. Things to notice after the first attunement 57
12. What is clearing 61
13. How to access Reiki 67
14. The Reiki balance 73
15. Using Reiki for distance healing 81
16. Self-healing 85
17. The chakras 89
18. Additional positions utilizing one or more chakra 99

Reading List 101
Bibliography 105
About the Author 109

~

~ Foreword ~

Today I will not worry.
Today I will not anger.
Today I will honor all others.
Today I will earn my living honestly.
Today I will be grateful.

-- Susan Caldwell

~ Introduction ~

Anything and everything stated in this workbook is from the experience of Susan Caldwell. It is meant to give you, the reader, the student of Reiki, guidelines. Accept and reject at your own discretion. Follow your own truth, your path. Be true to your Source and yourself above all else.

The information in this book references healing which is a different discipline than traditional Western medicine. I, in no way, offer medical advice or wish to discredit the medical community in any way. In case of serious illness always consult your physician. If you are adding Reiki to your health care program, please advise your physician.

I will interchange the titles Source, Universe, God, Spirit, Creator throughout this document. As Reiki has no religious connections, the energy used is the Source of Life. I mean to connect with no particular religion here, however, my background is Christian, and I do not deny my basis and strength in this particular dogma. I mean no offense in any words or lack of wording. I believe Source to be above religion and inclusive of ALL, all that is life. I believe we all are one and come from one Source.

~ 1 ~
Blessing the monetary exchange

As I am one with God, I am one with my God, for God is both the
Giver and the Gift. I cannot separate the Giver from the Gift.
Shin, *The Game of Life and How to Play It* 94.

In our society we place value on something that is important to us and our life choices. The value of the exchange is measured typically by money. It is an honor for me to accept money in exchange for this Reiki II attunement. When the money is blessed for mind, body, and spirit it brings all aspects together for the betterment, the goodness, and the highest exchange for all concerned.

The student offering money verifies their choice to learn Reiki, to awaken to becoming a more loving person, to be more in control of his or herself, and to grow spiritually on their unique journey.

In turn, the Reiki Master/Teacher exchanges their knowledge and perspective, their understanding, and gifts through Reiki. Because of the attunement lineage, this exchange filters through each, and every, Reiki student/teacher.

I will barter a partial payment with a Reiki attunement but not the entire price. I believe the ingrained value of money has an aspect that cannot be ignored. And I do not wish for money to hinder or stop a person's desire to learn. I will say that 95% of the Reiki attunements I have gifted, Reiki is not used or practiced by that recipient!

When the person hands me the payment, I hold it in my hands in a prayer position and ask that the money return to them tenfold. I provide a vase or jar to place the money in for the rest of the class.

I then welcome each student to the highest of their unique and individual good. To learn. To co-create. To be the best their Creator meant them to be. By saying yes with love to Reiki, I the student, honors his or herself, the teacher, and the planet.

THANK YOU, the reader, for inviting me to join you and to guide you on this occasion and in this sacred connection of our journeys.

For the goodness and glory for ALL concerned.

~ 2 ~
Welcome to Reiki.

"May the force be with you."
Yoda, *Star Wars*

One of the toughest things to do is try to describe Reiki. It is all about energy. Describing the energetic life force is not something that is in our everyday conversation. We search to establish and create a description to fit the slot for the "meaning of life" without the foundation of understanding what the rudimentary vital force is. So, we are climbing a ladder that is set on soft ground. The attempts to define Reiki without having a strong knowledge of energy is difficult. We are a species evolving, adapting, and reacting to the climatic and cultural situations we create.

Descartes said "I think, therefore I am." His reasoning cycles back into first believing in a Creator. Many thought patterns come back to faith which brings us to question the exact how, what, and why, that is our life force.

Is God just energy? Is the creative force of life a God? Each of us will have to answer these questions as they arise in our own exploration process. What is this phenomenon we call Life about? As we grow, getting in touch with a force that empowers us to examine and control ourselves can help us establish a more absolute grip on the how, what, when, where and why of what this thing called life is all about.

Determining some of the structural fundamental concepts is what Reiki is all about. It is a vibrational frequency of energy that is specific to making wellness possible on the physical, mental, emotional, and spiritual levels. It is an energy frequency that has an intelligence beyond what we can grasp. Is it faith healing? Yes. Faith healing with an intelligence and a sensory understanding and grasp of the faith force.

Often the words themselves are perceived as a woo- woo esoteric concept that evokes images of a Spiritual Guru. We search for a quick and precise explanation that is easy to understand.

Life is energy and Reiki is a frequency of that energy that supports the body's functions and helps the body heal itself. I am trained to draw the energy through me which helps others heal themselves.

Living in a world of noise and chaos causes stress and fatigue. Reiki relaxes and smooths the body's internal energy flow like a focused meditation with healing as the intention. It is Spirit infusing the physical to bring the original intent of healing into lives that are bombarded by outside forces.

Yet how does one explain the feelings and the healing that take place through the palms of a Reiki practitioner's hands? In simple terms: It is. It does. Faith in the feelings. Faith in the results. Faith in the connection.

Do you have to explain it at all? Ask the curious person to trust you and allow you try Reiki with them. Let them experience and then discuss.

Reiki is growing the life force within each person. And because Reiki encourages growth, whether it is through physical healing or an emotional release that gives understanding of our patterns, it gives us an inner strength to explore the meaning and processes of our lives.

In Touch with Reiki I

Blocks cause us to stumble and fall. As any blocks from fear, pain, or misunderstanding fall away, we adapt to what comes next into our life. As a result, we begin to learn some of the why we are here, how we fit, what our purpose is.

As we shed blocks, we become lighter energetically. We expand our understanding of the "who, what, when, where and why" we are here and how we fit with those around us and the situations we find ourselves in.

If the life force is strong enough the blocks will fall away, and the explanations will come.

Reiki is. One needs to feel it to believe it. Try it. If it does not work for you move on to something else. If it works for you study it, use it, play with it, and heal yourself from the inside out. Grow in the beauty that is you. The wonder that is unique to YOU.

Whatever path brought you here, I look forward to sharing this extraordinary phenomenon with you. Know that Reiki has found you and whether or not you use the energy for self-healings or you choose to study further and become a practitioner or teacher, your life will change.

Einstein postulated that all matter is energy, and that this energy is in constant motion, some at higher speeds than others. As physical beings we exist within this universal moving rhythm, the pulsing heart, the intake and release of breath. So, what defines the basics, the structure of those movements? Energy. Energy = life.

Everything is energy. Life is energy. Opening yourself to Reiki allows an increased flow of this life force energy. It brings us into greater harmony with our being and closer in touch with our Source. A Reiki attunement gives you increased connection and the ability to call on that energy at your own bidding. What does this mean? It means that if you invite the Reiki-intensified energy into your physical form, your life force becomes stronger and the vibrational levels that connect you with the earth's force rise.

If you think of your body as a unit of transportation, as a housing unit for the soul -- then honoring yourself is an act of honoring the life force that propels the physical, mental, and emotional layers.

Life is energy. Every single thing is composed of energy, the force from which we are born, exist in and to which we return. Some people relate this to an increased spiritual connection leading back to an all-powerful, All-in-One, God-type origin. Thus, the connections between spirit and earth are fine-tuned, bringing you closer to nature, fellow humans, animals, every object, or thing which has energy. Think about that for a bit.

> Everything. Every thing.
> Every single thing.
> Everything big and small,
> through every doorway,
> and down each hall.
> And you are integral to it all.

Reiki realigns us with our Source, our Creator, with the life-giving energies inside ourselves, the All-There-Is. It clears out negatives while augmenting the positives of physical, emotional, and spiritual transactions.

Reiki is a life-line streaming light through the body's core warding off the darkness of separation from the Light of Creation.

Reiki allows a renewal with the Spirit of Being, the Creator.

To an open and willing spirit Reiki brings with it an ultimate, intimate knowledge/wisdom found within the Creator/Life Force. A

In Touch with Reiki I

Reiki practitioner becomes a conduit for the energy connection for anyone.

Reiki re-establishes a wholeness and a sense of well being.

Reiki gives rise to unconditional love, allowing for intensified contentment and peace.

Reiki is living in the present moment, unburdening ourselves from the past, gathering faith to attend to the unfolding and unknown future.

Reiki gives us the ability to see with greater understanding our unique connections with others, within ourselves, and into our soul's mission. With this energy flows a wisdom that is beyond our knowledge. The energy heals on all levels. Often, physical results are swift and easy to identify. But most times the dis-ease is released in layers, a "peeling off," so the body can adjust in stages and as the "work" progresses. Often emotional issues will arise for the client and for the practitioner to view. When these are released, often a sense of peace and well-being changes the person and the physical area.

Disease as we speak it and write it as one word can be sentencing and become baggage. Written with a hyphen the word is broken down into its parts. Dis means the absence of. Ease refers to "the condition of being comfortable or relieved, freedom from pain, worry or agitation" (The American Heritage College Dictionary 394, 431). Dis-ease then is the absence of comfort and so becomes much easier to work with in terms of energy release.

Reiki does not conflict with any medical treatment and will, perhaps, enhance and speed up healing processes. Speak with your doctor about how you are incorporating Reiki. Note your dosage of medicines, any changes and how the medicines work with the body in its new vibration.

There are many paths to wellness and Reiki will benefit and compliment other methods of healing. It will make herbs and oils more effective.

Reiki establishes a method of taking control of one's own body, bringing in Spiritual energy with which the body can heal itself.

Reiki is an invitation to give you back the strength of your essence. You will re-member as it reconnects you to the essence of who exists within your physical house, your body.

Some claim Reiki once was available as a birthright, that an attunement or initiation into the Reiki vibration was part of the rites of passage for all. Over time the importance of connection to this vibration lost its status and was almost lost to our knowledge. Reiki, however, is now making a resurgence through an increased number of attunements and practitioners. It is moving across the planet in a wave, like a lighthouse beacon whose beam gets brighter and stronger as it reunites people to their Source and to the life force connection we all have with ourselves, other people, places, and things.

Reiki is saying YES to the Universe so one can begin to better understand the choice and responsibilities of free will and co-creation.

Now that you have said yes to Reiki, universal connections called synchronicities or miracles will begin to happen in, around and through you that will amaze and dazzle. You will be more in touch with your own truth and your own mission and your own purpose here on this planet. Open yourself to these omnipresent connections. Be surprised and grateful at the gifts offered in this blossoming relationship between the spiritual and physical.

Reiki cannot cause harm. In every article, book, and with every practitioner I have talked to this guarantee is unanimous.

Reiki cannot cause harm.

Thank you for saying yes. I welcome and bless you as you embark on the world anew with Reiki.

Susan Rea Caldwell

~ 3 ~
New Reiki information

Reissuing the In Touch with Reiki I, II, and III Manuals for Students/Teachers gives me cause to reflect on the ever-growing importance of Reiki in my life, giving me an amazing sense of self-strength and capability to travel through the experiences of my life. Reiki is my lifeline, my anchor, my launch pad!

What I know is that Reiki supports any additional healing modality, enhances all innate talents, and gives support when looking at issues as an involved participant or as an observer. What I will share is how I learned to let go and allow the Reiki energy to flow and heal with its own wisdom.

One of my greatest lessons has been with my friend I will call Tomi. Tomi and I worked in a small doctor's office together as receptionists. She was diagnosed with breast cancer during her second pregnancy, age 27. It took this conservative Baptist woman a bit to say yes to my invitations to try Reiki, yet when she did, she loved the relaxation it brought her.

We did not have much time for Reiki as Tomi was a mother and wife, working full-time while struggling with chemo and radiation. We set up a twin bed in a spare room in the office where we would "work" in 15–25-minute stints on lunch hours and occasionally before 8am. With so limited time and space, I did not work the chakras or concern myself with any hand positions. I sat at the head of the bed with a pillow and Tomi's head on my lap. I worked with Archangel Gabriel because Tomi named the child she was carrying at the time of her diagnosis Gabriel.

As Tomi learned to relax into the energy, we would "disappear" into the healing process. I learned to completely trust the linear time passage because at the perfect time, every time, we would both come "back." The Reiki took her to a safe, pain free state of no fear. Until…Tomi began to feel the Reiki was causing her more pain when the session was over than the tranquil state was beneficial. I believe she began to leave her body during these sessions. I could not get her to understand that concept. I was conflicted, struggling to understand why the Reiki was hurting her and that I could no longer use it to help her through her illness and make the cancer go away. I stopped putting my directly hands on her and I began to send distance Reiki to her surroundings. And her condition continued to worsen.

As I struggled with all this, a colleague told me that by putting my hands on Tomi's head where the cancer had metastasized, I was feeding the cancer. I completely freaked out until after much research, prayer, and many consultations with other energetic healers and Reiki practitioners, I became, and continue to be, 100% convinced that Reiki cannot do harm. My intentions for her healing were pure. They were colored by my egoic desire, a human limitation embossed with much love for my friend. I believe the energy does what it is guided to do by the person receiving the energy and that neither my ego nor my belief system could interfere with that. And, I believe I am forgiven, excused, and blessed, as I continue to learn and grow in understanding the nature of Reiki energy and of living without trying to control and/or judge.

My lesson in this was twofold. First, it was my adamant desire, hope, prayer, wish, and intention that Tomi regain perfect health. I believe this is what she wanted, and I believe she took her life contract to the foot of God to plead her case. She wanted to stay and raise her children, do her job, live this lifetime. It was not to be. And, I had to completely let go of the outcome and allow Tomi her relationship with her experience; not judge God; keep my own faith, not only in God, but faith in my own energetic capabilities and limitations.

As a result of that experience, I have decreased the number of hand positions I use during most of my healing sessions. Because people allow themselves so little down time and put themselves under so much pressure, I like for them to be as quiet and still for as long as possible. So, I have them lie face up on the table the whole session, no longer having them turn over to work on their back chakras.

First, I place my hands under the person's head for, sometimes, 30 minutes of the whole session. I cup their skull with my fingers at the base of their skull. So often headaches are felt here, and stress so easily finds its way here. Fingers pressing on the base of the skull is, well, my two-year client says, is the very best and moans her discontent every time I take my hands away, no matter how long I have stayed on this position! She says she feels the energy working through her whole body from this position and is able to connect with it.

Then I move to their side and place one hand under the person's neck and the other under the base of their spine. I call this the cradle position. To lie in it feels like you are wrapped in warmth, love, and safety. I believe this position works in all the chakras. If I find one or another chakra needs attention, I can blow the symbols or healing into it. Or I can use my eyes to send healing, or I ask my guides to handle that spot.

Next, I will hold the adrenals to release toxins by placing one hand just under their hip and the other on their side almost like my hands are in a 90-degree angle. Many people do not like their belly touched but touching their side seems to be okay. I will often switch hands at the same position to refill any energetic release with healing Reiki.

Then I hold the relaxed person's feet to ground them back in. If they have gone deep into the session, I will brush their legs, physically touching them, from the knees to the feet, three or four times. Then I do the usual aura sweeping. I tap them on the shoulder to let them know the session is complete. I leave the room to cleanse my hands to they can fully "return." I bring them a glass of water to remind them that drinking plenty of water further facilitates the healing over the next few days.

At one point in my Reiki career (for many years) I wanted to know, see, and/or hear the energies at work. I wanted to understand what the person was releasing, how it was affecting their body. After all, lots of my companions could see it, feel it, hear it and I wanted to, too! But I don't. Yet, I have grown to be very content in accepting my personal gifts. I believe I am most competent when I completely step out of the way of the process, disappear into the moment, and let the energies do their calling. It is simply my responsibility to be the most clear and unbiased Reiki channel I can be.

The Reiki process is between the energy and the receiver! And I am finally content and confident in allowing that to happen and simply being a part of the moment.

I encourage you to respect and honor the unique and individual Reiki practitioner that you are and that you will grow into. Be your blessed self and accept your uniqueness.

~ 4 ~
How Reiki works

"Only when we can devote ourselves without being prejudiced by our thoughts and feelings, will we become an instrument for the universal life energy."
Petter, *The Original Reiki Handbook of Dr. Mikao Usui* 21.

The concept of Reiki energy in our goal-oriented show-me society, seems abstract almost to the point of disbelief. Can we touch energy? Can we see what gives us life? Can we hear energy? Yes. So, doesn't it stand to reason that when the energy becomes sluggish, life is not as vibrant? Doesn't it stand to reason we would want to define and understand and manipulate the energy for our own well-being and contentment?

If energy is the component life is derived from, then doesn't it stand to reason that disconnection from this energy will cause stress, illness or pain? When times were simpler, when technology did not overshadow our lives, we were more in tune with nature and the energy that makes up our being. As we lose touch with this natural alliance we suffer. Reiki reconnects. It realigns and strengthens any misaligned connections. Reiki enhances, opens us to the central energy source that has become fuzzy, unclear, and out of focus. It opens us to a renewed sense of life and of life's purpose. Reiki reaffirms our state of being.

The body operates in an electromagnetic grid system. This system looks much like the body layered in sheets of graph paper. Lines run up and down the body and through the field around the body which is called the aura or the electromagnetic field.

Energy is drawn into the body via chakras. There are seven major chakras or energy centers located in the central core of the body from the root to the crown. These centers draw energy into the body specific to their location. They also relate to certain emotional and spiritual concerns in relation to their physical location. The seven primary chakras are located on the front and back of the body. They must function at an optimum level to discourage dis-ease and discomfort. There are many other secondary chakras. (See the chapter on chakras, pg 35.)

The physical body is often the end recipient of many of our "problems," and because of our lack of knowledge about the connections of mind, body and spirit, the physical becomes the primary frame of reference for measuring success or failure in healing.

Yet, the physical is not always where the healing energy will be focused. Reiki has an intelligence, a wisdom which overrides our own limited wisdom, and physical symptoms may not be the first ones the Reiki energy chooses to attend to. So, if a physical symptom is not alleviated during a balance, then perhaps an emotional issue or a spiritual issue has been attended to. Trust that the energy is going to the place where it will work for the highest and best good. As Reiki is utilized the body's energy field becomes lighter and will no longer be capable of holding as much negative or harmful "stuff."

So, just what is a block? An energy block is created when we take on trauma of any sort. Trauma can be from any thought, word, action, or deed that we take into our multi-layered being. It can be a thought, word, action, or deed we are responsible for initiating or from someone else that we have decided to accept as our truth.

One way not to do this is to follow the guidelines of Don Miguel Ruiz in his best-selling book The Four Agreements. The four are:

In Touch with Reiki I

Be Impeccable with your word.
Don't take anything personally.
Don't make assumptions.
Always do your best.

But we do take things on. We take words from other people, most often the hurtful ones and the ones that hit our issues of self-worth and confidence, into ourselves. These create blocks in the grid of our energy system. When we allow someone to hurt our feelings or when we bang our shin on a table, we allow something that is not loving to exist in our field. This is a block.

Blocks can also stem from outside sources. Walking through a negative field like a room where there has been a conflict or sitting with a person who is very negative and angry can leave negative debris in our field. We live in a world that slams us with negativity from the news to the personal beliefs about good and bad luck as seen by the victim mentality and the masses of litigious lawsuits of blame. We have polluted the planet. We live fast and furious, and the energy gets chaotic, and people get chaotic with it, creating more chaos and the vicious cycle spins. The way to control the spin for you is to recognize the situation for what it is, get out of the chaos, and find a safe place. Imagine the dramas as a storm and you in the calm center or the eye.

Reiki will facilitate this process. As you work with the energy you will be able to take yourself with a greater sense of peace and safety into the many situations that exist around you. As your blocks are cleared, your own energy will run smoother as you become stronger and more capable of living harmoniously through the storms of life.

Also, as you live in greater harmony, others will aspire to do the same. You become a magnet and a mentor to others seeking inner peace as you live.

See blocks as dark and Reiki as light. Light eliminates darkness. With light, darkness is no more. So, it is with the blocks. As positive Reiki energy is brought into your system it pushes out the negative.

The recipient draws upon the energy. As a vessel you may let it flow without directive or you may ask it to attend to certain wanting or suffering areas.

Reiki's own directive guarantees a recipient will not receive too much Reiki or that the Reiki will, in any way, be harmful. Reiki energy is positive energy. The worst that can happen is that nothing will happen if a recipient refuses the energy.

Reiki is different from other healing modalities because it offers automatic protection from taking on another's negativity. The attunement process is also unique to Reiki and offers networking capabilities within a family tree, of sorts, to all involved.

Reiki is becoming more commonplace as more practitioners are attuned and are seeing the benefits in themselves and those they touch. Many large hospitals are including Reiki practitioners on staff and are offering Reiki to interested patients and family. As allopathic medical fields need scientific proof, perhaps this is an opportunity to share our gifts and understandings with them in love and appreciation while we, in return, honor their gifts and understandings and methods of healings.

Marilyn Schlitz, Ph.D., director of research at the Institute of Noetic Sciences and senior scientist at the Geraldine Rush Cancer Research Institute at the California Pacific Medical Center in San Francisco, says, in her article in the June 2003 issue of Spirituality and Health, "the world really is coming together, fast. While tension continues between those who believe that the healing system can be reduced to biological processes and those who seek to involve a more holistic and far-reaching view of the healing system, it is clear that a new dialogue is emerging." (p12).

It is up to us as Reiki practitioners to use our talents and gifts to help those around us find theirs. Is it your mission to share goodness and health with others? Is it your mission to become a healer? You will know.

~ 5 ~
The history of Reiki

> We come to know Dr. Usui as a man not satisfied with surface appearances; one who would strive to embody the truths he had found. Furthermore, this was a man who dedicated his efforts to assisting others along the[ir] journey of discovery.
> Narrin, *One Degree Beyond* 84.

We work with stories and live the effects of stories and tales that cannot be proven or disproved over the course of the passing of time. And as much as the history of Reiki matters because it is our heritage, it does not matter as much as the conviction that what flows through our hands works.

The following is how I have bridged together the story from re-reading Diane Stein's Essential Reiki, Frank Arjava Petter's The Original Reiki Handbook of Dr. Mikao Usui and JaneAnne Narrin's One Degree Beyond.

Stein's text has been like a bible to me and those I have trained with. She is a warrior and a pioneer.

Narrin, in One Degree Beyond takes an interesting approach to humanizing Dr. Usui's journey to the discovery of Reiki energy methods. She weaves the tale of a pilgrim that gives us someone to reflect on and to mentor.

The Original Reiki Handbook of Dr. Mikao Usui describes

Frank Arjava Petters and his Japanese wife Chetna on their visit to Japan to uncover the mysteries of missing Reiki knowledge and connection. What they found was an active Japanese community that is not concerned about publicity. He also found Dr. Usui's tombstone and texts that detail a healing session, giving hand placements and methods of drawing in and identifying the energy. One important addition is the Gassho meditation to learn and strengthen the energy connection.

As a culture, we seem to enjoy creating heroes and unraveling the status we have given to them. Presidents fall from grace, as well as other political figures and business leaders. Athletic super achievers are exposed for transgressions the culture considers negative behavior. Or the above "get away with" things not acceptable for others. Priests and televangelists are defrocked in disgrace because their human characteristics grow bigger and stronger than their spirit connection. Extremists are represented in many factions and every religion. Open your eyes to what speaks to you in other people's behavior. Learn your truth through what troubles you about others. Know, above all, we are all souls here together having an imperfect, physical struggle. This includes the presidents, priests, and basketball players.

I suggest you research Reiki and energy healing and the spiritual path you are walking until you are satisfied. Then add your own views to those already out there. Write and print your own book. Let us all contribute our viewpoint with love and without judgement in an effort to promote tolerance for all.

Your knowledge as well as the knowledge of the other people will increase as you dig further into your own belief systems and as more viewpoints are brought to the discussion table.

The history of Reiki is a convoluted story. Most recollections will tell you Dr. Usui was a curious spiritual seeker who wanted an answer to the question, "How did the ancient healers heal?" The most common tale says that he traveled extensively, leaving Japan, searching and researching, that he attended a theological school in Chicago, went back to his home country and visited a monastery at Mt. Kurama where he was invited to read the ancient texts. (Petter calls it Mt. Kurma. Stein calls this place Mt. Koriyama. I choose to use Mt Kurma because Petter visited Japan and his text is the more recent of the two.) He did not find his answer. He went to the top of Mt. Kurma, considered a very holy place, and prepared to meditate and sit with his concerns. He marked the passing of days by using rocks. On the 21st day he had a vision. The vision was the Reiki symbols and the method of Reiki healing. He left the mountain and four miracles happened. One was when he stumbled and injured his toe, and it was healed when he placed his hands on it. The second is when he ate without getting sick after a 21-day fasting period. The third was the healing of a toothache of a young lady who lived in the house where he stopped to ask for food. The fourth miracle was when he placed his hands on the monk who was in bed with a severe arthritis attack at the monastery where Dr. Usui was living.

Dr. Usui took his gifts to the streets of Kyoto and began to work with people who were grateful but who came back again and again with the same illnesses. He was healing the physical, but clients were not addressing the emotional or spiritual aspects. Dr. Usui began to travel and became a pilgrim walking the roads of Japan until he met Chujiro Hayashi. They opened a clinic where they set up an exchange of goods for services. He began to teach Reiki to others in the clinic and to create new Reiki Masters.

Hawayo Takata, in Hawaii, was ill with gall bladder problems and her body was too weak for surgery. She visited her parents in Tokyo and was treated with Reiki at a clinic. Over a period of two years, she was given enough Reiki healing to eliminate her symptoms. She taught and attuned to two levels of Reiki.

In 1938 Hayashi traveled to Hawaii and passed Takata her Master level attunement. They did a lecture tour together.

When Hayashi visioned World War II and being called to join the Japanese armed forces, he chose to transition. But first he called Takata, and she traveled to Japan and was named his successor. Stein and others state that the clinic was destroyed and Takata became the sole surviving person on the planet with Reiki knowledge and training. She began teaching and training by word of mouth. There were no written texts, no recordings of the symbols. Before she died in December 1980, she had trained 22 Reiki masters. Takata did not allow her students to take notes. She required a long-time commitment and lots of money for the third/Master level attunement. The reasoning was to keep the lineage pure and to protect the Master level for those committed to the study and sacredness of Reiki energy. She felt the symbols were too sacred to travel outside the classroom and she often changed the structure of the symbol according to the student.

It is in Takata's writings that Dr. Usui's connection with Western theological doctrine is spoken of. Few writings or Reiki books state that connection. According to William Rand there is no record of Dr. Usui attending or receiving a degree from the University of Chicago Divinity School.

Along comes Diane Stein, seeker, energy healer, feminist, and practicing Wiccan who is drawn to study Reiki in her pursuit of understanding energy and its manipulation for healing. Stein found her journey to attaining three levels of Reiki very difficult. I find her tenacious search for healing methodologies much akin to Dr. Usui's!

Stein was directed by her own Spirit Guides to persevere and study and to publish the Reiki symbols. From a non-traditional stance, I believe Stein has opened a path to making Reiki energy available to many. However, her historic decision has created much controversy and discontent in the Reiki community causing a rift between traditional and non-traditional factions.

In Touch with Reiki I

In studying the history of Reiki, read everything you can about Dr. Usui. Read his texts and piece together his story remembering he was a remarkable and determined man who went before us and brought to our use a remarkable system of healing that can bring peace to the traumas that burden us in this physical body.

I take counsel from many areas of Dr. Usui's story. I feel an admiration for the determination and tenacity he showed in his search. The 21 days of meditation is a model for being still and listening and waiting for the answer, clearing ourselves of all our own directives - being a clear vessel so that the spirit message can come through true and unfettered.

The first four healings are recorded in all the texts I have read. Interestingly, the first two healings may just be the toughest for us to adhere to: self-healing. Dr. Usui injured his toe. A metaphysical translation of that injury would mean his fear of going forwards, and perhaps stumbling, with his new information and any concerns he had with presenting it to the world. I translate this to mean his fear surfaced and I see that he put his hands down, attended to the matter and was able to walk on. If Dr. Usui had ignored his toe, and had no self-knowledge of the capabilities of Reiki healing, would his words and his enthusiasm have been as effective when working with others? Physician heal thyself.

How much credence can others place in one who is not working on her/himself? Do you want to hire a plumber whose home is riddled with broken pipes? Do you aspire to the words of a preacher who is full of vitriol?

Dr. Usui's second occasion for healing also involved his own physical body. He ate without physical repercussions after a 21-day fast. His body accepted the food and he fed himself so that he could move on! I suspect he used the symbols to bless the food so that it did not cause trauma to a weakened body.

Taking nourishment in the physical sense, he was strong enough to move forward. Respect for one's own physical body are the first two recorded healings. Think about it.

The third healing opportunity came with the young woman in the home where Dr. Usui was fed. She had a toothache. He facilitated healing so she was able to chew and take in nutrition. Was this need for sustenance on the physical, or on the emotional, mental, and spiritual level? When her toothache was "fixed" the healing touched all levels, I suspect. Imagine the joy, wonder and celebration in the household at the experience!

The fourth opportunity came when Dr. Usui got home. A monk he lived with suffered with arthritis. Arthritis is stiffness, aches, and discomfort within the body's movement capabilities. In metaphysical terms it is feeling victimized, being self-critical and self-destructive (Bourbeau 377). This fits with Reiki possibilities in our lives, doesn't it?

Opportunities to use your Reiki like those that came to Dr. Usui will come to you also. Tracker was my miracle opportunity. A lanky, bow-legged beagle with a heart as big as the state and no manners. She got on the dining room table for the saltshaker, once! Tracker was a runaway who made a home in the rusted-out car on the farm just above my friend's property in Southern Ohio. She had seven puppies and was starving. My friend found her and fed her. We took the puppies to the pound and returned the next morning to re-rescue them!

After we got her fed and stronger, she developed a nasty skin infection. Over the course of 6-8 months, we took turns housing her for weeklong periods, nursing and Reiking her. She had ear mites and fleas, a weird something on her mouth. She had arthritis from having both front legs broken. We would Reiki her, nurse her and then she would get something else. When she recovered, she was wild and had to return to the country to live. Eight years later she was still tracking and hobbling on those bowlegs and being her sweet, Beagle self.

Tracker helped us learn about the feel of energy in our hands and how it flowed into different parts of Tracker's body. We learned about patience in the healing process and how to let go of the outcome of the process. We learned that Reiki works because of that little dog who ate corn off the cob as smooth as an Underwood manual typewriter, chomping line by line with her little front teeth.

Tracker gave back to us a sense of humor, that energy work could be fun and not just a call-in-the-Gods state of being. She gave us hope because of her tenacity. She lived in the now and accepted what was offered her. She proved someone would be just around the corner to pick us up every time we fell! She gave us authenticity.

Getting back to the many lessons of the Dr. Usui story. Money. Tracker didn't pay us money, but the lessons she gave us were worth much more. Money is not the be all and end all, but exchange is important. The value you place on the exchange will bring up many issues and it is discussed often in the many published Reiki texts and here in the chapter Blessing the Monetary Exchange. Do you want to make a living using your Reiki? Then you need money to live. It is the currency of exchange we have set up here on this planet. If you would like to barter, then barter. Remember the balance. And remember the time you have spent studying and working on yourself. A painter builds into his price the cost of all his education and practice, and he builds to the moment of the current canvas. Your dedication to the art of healing counts. Honor yourself and respect the time and effort you place in this healing endeavor.

If the energy of the exchange is unbalanced, you will know it. Trust me. Your life force energy is not going to let you walk away from this one without some resolution!

The history of Reiki brings up racial issues. I think it is interesting that the energy comes to the west from Japan, our World War II enemy. The bitter war wounds overlapping with the economic foreign imports challenges during the 70s and 80s create an interesting dichotomy. Healing and war and economic struggle. Are we hereby presented situations by Spirit for healing?

These cultural biases were once a part of the difficulties I faced in sharing Reiki knowledge when I was a new practitioner. The concept and the background were foreign, strange, not in line with the European-English tradition my Appalachian heritage accepted or understood.

In addition, I am a writer, a communicator and, guess what I could not do? Easily explain Reiki. How does one communicate the what, who, when, where or how of something so esoteric? Talk about frustrating. Chalk that up to one of the issues incorporated in my clearing! And note how this is a prime example of how Reiki works to heal the planet one person at a time.

The Dr. Usui story also spotlights gender issues. Dr. Usui did not attune females. His culture is renowned for its often cruel patriarchal structures. Dr. Hayashi, however, did attune his wife and Mrs. Takata. A woman then became responsible for the spread of Reiki in America – Mrs. Takata, a woman from Hawaii, a state whose cultural background is considered tribal and a giant step outside the traditional Anglo-American heritage.

Reiki brings to the table many issues that at its very core addresses the meshing of traditional and new. Add the Buddhism and you have religion. Issues? Dare I postulate that religious intolerance has caused more death on this planet than disease or famine or natural disasters?

So, the very essence of Reiki becomes a way of healing religious conflicts via energy - pure life force energy. For WE ARE ALL

In Touch with Reiki I

ONE. We are taking part, an active part, in healing the ills of this planet by using Reiki energy. We are making ourselves available to contribute our time and efforts to helping others help themselves and heal—one person at a time.

For years in Appalachia people have been practicing hands-on healing. They experience faith healing. They are safe in their church giving all the credit to the Lord.

Warts are "charmed" off. Spirits are seen, heard, and felt. My girlfriend's mother could cure the croup with her breathe. It was not to be spoken of, though. Children were brought to the back door in the dark of the night and thanks were whispered.

In my neck of the woods, touch therapy is not new, but calling it Reiki and studying it is. Miracles and healings can and do happen and we, as energy workers, can choose to participate in them with a more learned knowing and understanding, co-creating our universe. We are not puppets, but co-creators. I believe that Spirit wants us to learn to use more of what is true and pure in our lives and will send as much as we need, and as much as we ask for.

~ 6 ~
What makes Reiki different from other healing modalities?

The attunement process makes Reiki different. It creates a lineage, a web of connections. It is a universal understanding that we can tap into. It also means that we have learned this technique from someone else's study via their direct connection. Reiki is not something that can be learned from a book at home. It is a family, a connection energy. This binds us with a stronger and brighter energy thread.

Reiki uses sacred symbols that represent healing vibrational frequencies that work parallel to specific areas of trauma. Their use gives a practitioner additional tools with which to work through their own blocks and those of the person under their hand.

Reiki comes with automatic protection from taking on another's negativity. It provides a confidence in knowing that whatever another person's stuff is, it will not hinder or hurt us. We as volunteers in channeling energy can rest assured that the same energy that heals will protect and guide us. Reiki energy is all inclusive and works on all levels of the healing process which is the greatest benefit and special attribute of Reiki. Reiki heals both the healer and the healee at the same time. There is an automatic give and take, an immediate response to the adage "what you give out returns to you," or to put it in Biblical terms, you reap what you sow.

Visualize yourself as a pipeline. If your pipe is corroded with old belief patterns and fears, then where is the healing going to take place? The first place it finds a need. So, clearing yourself of hindrances on all levels assists the others you put your hands on.

Reiki becomes a way of life, a way of looking at every situation that you find yourself in. It is a belief system that strengthens because it is loving, healing, and rewarding.

~ 7 ~
The Raku

The Raku is a symbol received in the third Usui attunement. There are those who may disagree with my publishing this symbol in a first level Reiki manual without the attunements and teachings of further steps in Reiki. I include a description of it here because of chaotic energies in the world and because people are becoming more aware of energy patterns and are becoming more susceptible to the energy fields around them. As a result, it can become more difficult to separate what is ours from what is someone else's. The Raku will help. It separates.

The lightning bolt will separate and create a boundary between you and another person or energy you do not wish to incorporate into yours. For example, if there is a store you do not like to go into or a room, draw the Raku in front of your heart before entering and you will not feel the incompatibility as harshly. If there are people, places, things which you believe drain your energy, draw the Raku. It will disconnect and separate.

If you are pushing the grocery cart or on the bus feeling uncomfortable, draw the Raku in your palm chakras. Visualize it between you and whatever you are uncomfortable with – a violent scene on the TV, or a disgruntled neighbor.

Susan Rea Caldwell

~ 8 ~
The Reiki principles

Just for today, do not anger.
Just for today, do not worry.
We shall count our blessings and honor our fathers and mothers,
our teachers and neighbors and honor our food.
Make an honest living.
Be kind to everything that has life.
Hawayo Takata, *The History of Reiki as Told by Mrs. Takata*

Just for today do not worry.
Just for today do not anger.
Honor your parents, teachers, and elders.
Earn your living honestly.
Show gratitude to everything. Respect the oneness of all life.
Diane Stein *Essential Reiki*

Just for today, I will live in the attitude of gratitude.
Just for today, I will not worry.
Just for today, I will not anger.
Just for today, I will do my work honestly.
Just for today, I will show love and respect for every human being.
Paula Horan, *Empowerment Through Reiki*

These are beautiful words we all can aspire to. They remind us to live in the now, to love all of life. It is so simple and yet it is so difficult at times. Live from moment to moment and if you fall off the love-everything wagon, work towards forgiving yourself and all others involved and move on. Just for today. Just for the moment, because this moment is all we have.

~ 9 ~
The process of the first attunement

An Attunement is a ceremony of opening and empowering your physical body to accept and then be able to transfer Reiki energy. In the process the crown, heart, and palm chakras are opened to connect you to the flow of the Universal Life Force through your physical body.

Passing attunements is an honor given to Reiki practitioners who have attained the Master III level. This personal transference is one of the features that makes Reiki unique to the modalities of hands-on therapy. By the passing of attunements, the student is connected to the Teacher/Master who is in turn connected as a student and Master by way of lineage. Reiki becomes analogous with family, a heritage with established traditions, creating an auric, energetic bond between all those involved.

Be it an organized ceremony or a brief answer-to-Spirit calling, the attunement process focuses on one thing: opening the recipient to the flow of Reiki energy. The Reiki Master visually opens the aura of the recipient, draws and blows the sacred Reiki symbols through the crown chakra down to the heart and then into the palms of the hands and up through the heart chakra. The aura is then closed and an additional symbol for separation is drawn down the back.

Symbols are used in every culture and are representations of specific objects. Symbols are maps that lead to specific territories. For example: chair is a group of alphabetic symbols referring to a device used to sit in. The function of the chair comes to mind; however, the type of chair can vary from dentist to folding to reclining. Symbols are used in chemistry (H2O) and in literature (the red rose referring to love). Logos are symbols used by marketing departments.

The Reiki symbols are sacred geometric representations that relate to certain vibratory frequencies which resonate to specific aspects of healing. One symbol calls to the vibratory level of emotional healing. One symbol draws to it a more concentrated flow of energy. The act of placing the symbols in the auric field connects the recipient with those vibrations which allow the Reiki energy to flow through the body.

The recipient of an attunement may feel the energy coming through or may feel nothing. The sensations vary according to each individual. Some students will feel the symbols move and settle in. Some can feel the energy field opening. Many feel the presence of angels and guides. Some feel tired or exalted. Every range of emotion is possible. If one feels nothing it does not mean the attunement has not "taken." It simply means the person felt nothing! And that does not mean the attunement was not successful.

The Reiki Master giving the attunement also may feel nothing or something. This varies with the degree that the Master is in touch with the energy. Sometimes, but not always, I feel the aura opening and the new Reiki energy moving through. The intensity of these occurrences varies with the situation and the persons involved. I have felt the presence of ascended Reiki Masters who come to witness the ceremony. Angels and guides are always present. I have worked with Reiki Masters who see the symbols floating and penetrating the student's energy field.

Remember: There is everything spontaneous about attunements. They are individual. Each is unique. The beauty lies in the moment. It is the power of the now! Do not wish for a situation different than how it is presented to you and the special gift that you are. Honor

In Touch with Reiki I

the moment and the specific beauty of each blessed event.

I believe it is important to give newly attuned hands the opportunity to experience channeling Reiki. I put every new Reiki I person on the table in a round robin of sorts with all the students participating in and receiving a healing. This way the student has an opportunity to feel the energy and experience an energy balance. The healing process formulates an atmosphere for questions and gives the student some confidence in their ability to channel Reiki energy through their physical bodies. It also gives space for familiarizing new students with chakras and hand placements. Using the energy will ground the person and revitalize them if the attunement process has caused any energy drains.

To the new Reiki practitioner, I urge you to use your Reiki. Trust it. Enjoy it.

~ 10 ~
The first attunement

The first attunement is like a plugging in. It is an opening and an awakening to Life Force Energy. It enhances and encourages beneficial energy flow. The first attunement opens you to new levels of sensory feelings and images. It brings with it a more confident way to identify Spirit and the way Spirit moves within your life. It puts you more in tune with yourself. It provides a sturdy and steadfast core which empowers, supports, and stabilizes you no matter what the circumstance. It is a knowledge to hold on to, to build on, and to fall back on. It is an inner peace, a confidence, and a trust. It is a self-perpetuating love which flows through all living things. You are a lamp that is now plugged in.

The first attunement primarily allows for the ability to self-heal. Reiki is about loving yourself and forgiving yourself. The ability to lay hands upon another is also possible, but the first attunement focuses on building, loving, and healing oneself.

The new vibratory level of your body accepting Reiki into your energetic field will work from the inside out causing change first through a clearing and then by how you relate to the world around you. Reiki brings with it a more loving viewpoint and creates a deeper understanding of the Universal Life Force that connects us all. This greater understanding will cause extraneous energies to affect you and you will need to learn to adapt.

This self-focus is one that we often find difficult because we are taught that doing for oneself is selfish, that sacrifice and giving is what we are supposed to do. Giving to the point of depletion is, unfortunately, viewed as model behavior in this busy, accomplishment driven society. Yet how and what can we give if our strength is depleted? Can your car run without gasoline? Can an empty vessel pour blessings? No. What are the instructions for donning the O2 masks in an airplane? Put your own mask on first. You cannot help anyone else if you cannot breathe. With more time, love, and energy designated to the self, the self has more fuel, stamina, and wisdom to utilize and pass on. As you heal, remember, your beacon will shine brighter, missioning and beckoning to others.

Live by example. You have volunteered to live more in tune with your spiritual directives. Grab hold of your new strength and go forward with gusto.

Of course, Reiki energy can also be conveyed to animals and plants, to machines and situations. Dogs and cats love Reiki and are excellent practice vessels. Plants will wiggle with the energy transference. Dead hot water heaters may come back to life!

The strength of Reiki's influence and inspiration is unlimited if you are creative in your usage. One practitioner started a dead car battery with her Reiki. It fixed the monitor on my computer. It eliminates pain from burns, relieves cramps, lowers racing blood pulses. It is miraculous at relieving stress by bringing a sense of peace, trust, and overall well-being. You can change your environment with spiritual energy. Yes, you can!

Reiki cannot cause harm. In every article, book, and with every practitioner I have talked to this guarantee is unanimous. Reiki cannot cause harm.

USE YOUR REIKI. The more you use it the stronger it will flow, the more confident and knowledgeable you will become. The world needs healing. It happens one person at a time. As you are healed others around you will heal and you become the vessel by which you heal. Pass it on - one soul to another.

~ 11 ~
Things to notice after the first attunement

The experience of the attunement process varies from person to person. You may feel the symbols as they are passed to you. You may see colors flashing. You may experience enhanced feelings of peace, tranquility, or euphoria. You may feel nothing. Whatever it is, it is okay. The attunement will "take." I did have one student who claimed her attunement was not successful. I gave her another attunement. I have also done booster-like attunements if a student gets attuned and does not use the Reiki for whatever reason and wants to be refreshed. Any monetary concerns with this reattunement process would need to be discussed with individual Reiki Masters.

Hot hands. Your hands may tingle or warm like they do when they have been "asleep" and are just waking up. Allow yourself the moment to study and become aware of the physical sensations as you call Reiki to move through you.

Learned perceptions will further enhance future Reiki sessions because the language of Reiki is sensory.

Your hands may also run cold energy. And although warm is the most common, nothing is "wrong" with cold energy. Trust the knowledge of the Reiki. Giving up your judgments of how and why will increase the strength of your particular stream of Reiki.

Your hands may begin to channel Reiki long before your actual attunement at times when you least expect. In these cases, know that Spirit is calling to you. Honor and meet the directive by putting your hands where healing energy is needed. It may be on yourself, or on an animal, on a tree, a plant, or a friend.

Things, places, and people may not "feel" the same after your first Reiki attunement. This is Divine planning, and you should be attentive to these life changes. Your energy field is different now and may not fit where it did before. You may need to reconsider your thoughts, your concepts of things. You are now on a path to enlightenment, and you may need to adjust and adapt to the new ways.

If you are serious about changing your life and living your divine mission, I suggest you consider reading and following Shin's book The Game of Life and How to Play It. She has a powerful prayer called the Divine Plan. It will bring immediate and often drastic changes in your life as Spirit adjusts your life to meet your soul mission.

To state the Divine plan repeat, "Divine Love now dissolves and dissipates every wrong condition in my mind, body and affairs. Divine love is the most powerful chemical in the universe, and dissolves everything which is not of itself." (94). I always add that the process needs to be easy and graceful for everyone involved.

In addition to stating the plan, I advise reading the text to help you through this process. Be aware that this entreaty is serious and will bring QUICK changes to your life on all levels. And turning back is next to impossible.

Use your Reiki, even in 5-minute spurts. Be creative. Call on Reiki when you are driving (it will not hurt your car), in line at the grocery, in church, watching TV, reading, talking on the phone. The more you use it the stronger it becomes. The quieter you are with the application the more you will come to identify, understand, and feel comfortable with it.

Become aware of your own thought patterns. What do you say

to yourself in your mind chatter? How do you react to yourself and to others? With judgement? With criticism? With blame? Do you feel a victim or a co-creator in your universe? In situations that vex and confuse you ask yourself, "What would Love do?" And most importantly, learn to love yourself. You can be your best friend or your worst enemy. Make your choice. Forgiveness begins with self.

While washing my face one morning I found myself saying, "I'm bad to use soap on my face and not a facial cream." It is an expression I can hear my grandmother Hazel saying. "I am bad to..." Well, am I bad for using a bar of soap to wash my face? No, but I was standing right there looking in the mirror and telling myself it was so.

Reiki practitioners will get sick, but with the use of Reiki energy the symptoms should be less severe, and the 'bug' may move through your system faster. It is like a 24-hour virus in 12 hours. Some invasive things may slide past your energy field and no longer bother you. For example: A woman was prone to burning herself while cooking and using Reiki on the burns resulted in much less pain and quicker healing. With more intense emotional work she was able to discover why she kept burning herself. She hated cooking. She felt oppressed in the kitchen and felt she was getting "burned" by her family who did not recognize her abilities and sacrifices.

Wash your hands often and keep them well groomed. They are your representatives.

~ 12 ~
What is clearing?

Your commitment to use Reiki energy is to a new empowered self. Clearing with Reiki I will be your first step in realigning with your true energetic self. Like the kitchen drawer that has collected junk for years, your body has collected lots of junk. The junk causes the flow of energy to become constricted. These constrictions turn into dis-ease related symptoms. To shed these symptoms the body will go through some release processes or what is called "clearing." Clearing allows the life force energy to move easier and smoother through your system in the process of raising your body's vibrational level.

Clearing differs with each stage of Reiki. The first attunement will focus on physical issues, the second on emotional, and the third on spiritual. With each attunement the incoming energy will be magnified, intensifying the vibration in which you will exist and prompting the necessity to shed unwanted patterns.

No level of physical, emotional, or spiritual existence is affected apart from the other. But because of the power of the mind, emotion and spirit, the physical is the last place a trauma rests. So it is the place to begin when you start to unravel blocks stored in the energy system. The physical is, also, the area easiest to identify. As any physical symptoms abate the attached thought and belief patterns can also be addressed.

One level of Reiki is not a miracle cure for a disease that has taken years to develop, but never discount the validity of miracles.

A Course in Miracles says there is no order of difficulty in miracles (1.1.1 pg 3). Energy healing takes study and healing, as an ongoing process, involves all levels of mind, body, and spirit. Using Reiki can begin this process if you choose to engage in introspective spiritual endeavors. The degree to which Reiki affects you will depend on the degree to which you use and study it. Reiki I will, however, raise the body's vibration so that some of the less traumatic illnesses cannot find a place in your energy field to live. So, it offers some protection.

For 21 days subsequent to your attunement your body will clear to adapt to this new vibratory level. To learn and understand your new level of energetic flow, I encourage you to place your hands on one chakra a day for seven subsequent days beginning with the root chakra and moving up through the crown. I encourage you to repeat this very important cleansing cycle three times. This is to invite learning about the energy of who you are, to cleanse your blockages, and to keep your chakras open and functioning adequately. The 21-day process teaches and guides you into this new, life altering and beautiful world of self- healing.

I suggest doing complete self-healing two or three times a week during the three-week clearing process. If you have a Reiki partner, share Reiki balances. If there is a Reiki group that offers Reiki shares, attend them. (A Reiki share is when a group of practitioners get together to place the hands on themselves and others in a time of networking. It can be as elaborate as bringing potluck for dinner or a simple meeting in someone's living room. Each person gets a balance and is expected to put their hands down on the others.) This will lessen the effects of the clearing process and enlighten and ground you to Reiki ways and feelings.

Clearing is nothing to ignore. Clearing will "lighten your load." The blockages must work their way out of you in some physical or emotional process because they no longer fit in your vibratory pattern.

In Touch with Reiki I

Clearing may begin before the attunement and will vary with individuals. It may consist of a runny nose, diarrhea, and/or tiredness. You may have lots of gas, sweat more. One or any combination of these things will result as a physical manifestation of the body cleaning out the unwanted, the unnecessary. You will be cleansing a layer or so of anything which may prevent you from experiencing the Reiki energy to the highest level at this precise moment. Do not resent the discomfort; bless it as it leaves as you will become more free to run pure life-force energy.

If you are using your Reiki and drinking water the symptoms will not make you "sick." Clearing should not keep you from functioning in your usual activities. So, the diarrhea should not be accompanied by painful stomach cramps, or the runny nose with a cold. The symptoms are a result of your body cleansing itself. Enjoy the process of eliminating these physical blocks.

During the clearing you may find sensory images heightened to the point they may become overpowering. This should pass when the clearing process is over. Too much outside energy may become confusing and unsettling. Sounds that go on and on like Muzak or Blue Light Special announcements, "on hold" music or gas pump tunes may cause you distress. Blinking lights, neon or harsh fluorescent lights, the physical presence of crowds and traffic may become invasive and too intense for your comfort in this process.

I was in college as a returning student when I received all three levels of Reiki. We often went to a pizza place for lunch, but not during any clearing! The lights and sounds were way too intense, even though I was familiar with the place. Though I was with the same people I went with regularly, I could not sit and eat in the fluorescent lights and noise.

Honor yourself by protecting yourself from these interferences during your clearing. If the interferences become too much remember that you now have Reiki to protect you. Put your hands on yourself or on something and bring your Reiki through to balance and ground yourself.

You can now call Reiki to yourself at any moment for comfort. Sit with your hands in your pocket, with one hand on your leg. Go to a quiet place you like, breathe deeply, and relax in the healing energy you can now create.

I encourage you to stay inside your own familiar, protected environment as much as possible during these 21 days. Find time to be still, to meditate, to be with yourself. Take walks in nature. Allow yourself the peace of limited outside interference. Allow your spirit to flow free and open up to the loosened thoughts that have been locked away inside. Remember you are now more tuned into spiritual and universal connectedness that is unique and personal. Let go of any physical distress you hold onto. Let it surface and leave.

Reiki clearing may change some of your immediate social behaviors and also some habitual behaviors as well. Attunements make some people clean house, clean out drawers, the garage. Reiki clearing may be the cause behind many a yard sale! There arises this feeling of wanting organization and the need to move things out that are no longer needed or wanted. Any usual clutter becomes confining and limiting. Clearing returns one to the basics, to holding onto what is important and letting go of the rest.

This will hold true of emotional habits as well. If emotional issues surface, try to cleanse them also. I do not believe in coincidences. This is my own personal truth, not anything you should accept as yours if you do not relate to it. I believe everything happens for a reason, thus whatever events, thoughts, or people are brought to you during this time are brought to you and for you by Spirit as a gift. Do with them what you need to do to facilitate healing. Is the event created to give you an opportunity to learn true forgiveness and love, for yourself and others? Let the concerns surface. Do your best to deal with them and get clear of them. Deal with them knowing that you have the strength of Reiki to empower and support you and to heal you.

Unburden yourself from past behaviors, in particular the ones that can harm your physical body. Let Reiki assist you in uncloaking self-defeating habits. I quit smoking with the help of Reiki, putting my hands down when the cravings came.

Eat healthy foods during your clearing. I suggest eating as close to the ground as possible. Limit your intake of caffeine, sugar, and alcohol. Their effect will be intensified.

Water is healing and cleansing for the body and the aura. So extra baths or showers are ways of assisting you in the clearing process. Go swimming.

The clearing will happen whether or not you take an active role. The body will clear. Often people will feel the energy switch chakras at the 24-hour mark when the attunement took place. Some will be able to identify the issues presented in association with the chakra that is clearing. Some will not notice the changes.

If you feel physically out of balance, do twelve or so (always in even sequences) cross crawls. This is an exercise where you stand in place and lift the left arm and right leg (bent knee) followed by the opposite arm and leg. This will balance right and left sides.

If you feel mentally out of balance, place your hands on the front and back of the third eye chakra for several minutes. This will get your intuitive side running smoothly.

Breathe. Believe. Heal. Call your Reiki Master or someone you trust to discuss your feelings and concerns.

Drink water. The most common cause of headaches is dehydration. The toughest clearings seem to be a result of the person forgetting to drink water. The body will clear and if the "stuff" is not flushed out it hangs on with a vengeance making the symptoms more severe. Wash the surfacing stuff out. Let it go. Flush it out. Drink water.

The following are some of my student reactions after their first level attunement:

"On the drive home last Monday, I had all sorts of past "stuff" bubbling up from somewhere. I just built me an imaginary bonfire, took it out of the boxes, stuffed it all in trash bags and dumped it in the bonfire. Then, I thought, wait a minute, why am I keeping the boxes. I drug them out and tossed them in the fire, too!!!!"

"The peace I have felt since Mon. night is awesome! My life has been full of miracles and synchronicities since that night. The clearings I am doing are profound. I have been somewhat reclusive and tired, but I understand that is normal."

"I think I am getting more of a feel for how to heal myself. Moving my hands to where they are needed feels so natural How great to be driving in the car and placing one hand on the heart chakra and doing a clearing! I am writing my issues down as I had previously but now my desire to heal is much more intense. My angels and spirit guides are assisting my efforts.

"What a blessing Reiki is and I'm so happy you are part of my path. My sense of connection to life is so much greater...like Giving birth to a new me."

"I quit smoking. Lost the taste for cigarettes. I just can't light one!"

~ 13 ~
How to access Reiki

Your intention is enough to bring the Reiki through you. Your body may react by producing hot, oven mitt hands, or you may "sort of" feel the energy. You may feel nothing.

Trust that the energy is moving through you and that with continued use and experience you will become adept to the feel and sense of it. State your intention to do so. "I am confident in understanding energy."

For months after my first level attunement I repeated, "I am a competent and worthy Reiki healer."

To call on the Reiki, ask it to flow. "Reiki on."

State your intentions. "My intention is to heal on all levels of mind, body and spirit."

Remove yourself from all judgement. "My intention is that this energy be used for the highest and best good for all concerned."

When you finish with the healing ask the energy flow to cease. "Reiki off. Thank you, Spirit Guides, for your presence and direction and support."

I believe each of us has a Healing Guide that oversees us. In most of the Reiki literature they are called Spirit Guides. They are entities who volunteer to help with our healings. Yours will assist and guide you. They are a part of the intuition sensation involved in the healings. The person on the table also has an Angelic presence who will work with your Guides during healings. Even if you do not sense the presence of a healing Angel or Spirit Guide, know they are there for you and the situation. Our concepts are limited, but our Guides have the universal picture. The energy we channel brings with it this universal knowing and so for maximum use we, the practitioner, need to let go of the how, what, and why of it.

Although a Reiki attunement will protect you from taking on any negative release that may be associated with the healing of a client, you may want to establish a dialogue for protection to make yourself more comfortable. One mantra a Reiki Master uses is, "That nothing but good come from me and nothing but good come to me." Surround yourself with a symbolic shield of white light. A Glad bag of protection! If you are comfortable with using Christ energy, ask for the Light of Christ consciousness to surround you. This method brings a Christian, biblical resonance to using Reiki, but it is in my background. You are free to use or dismiss this as your heart directs whether or not you profess Christianity and/or a relationship with Jesus/Christ as part of your belief system.

Read, journal, study and meditate with the intention of developing a stronger relationship with your Guides. I believe they are anxious to work with us to facilitate as much healing as possible in every situation. Call on them. Speak to them. Respect and honor them.

Trust at all times during the healing that the energy is flowing, that your intention is being honored. "I am worthy. I am a loving Spirit." Find a mantra, sing a song. Know. Trust. Enjoy the exchange.

As Reiki energy is used you will become more accustomed to the feel, smell, and sound of it. You will become more comfortable identifying with it.

In Touch with Reiki I

Although you do not have to have meditative thoughts or any particular mental directive, I suggest you remove negative thought patterns while channeling Reiki. If negatives do come up (note recurring patterns), then maybe the Spirit Guides are trying to tell you to notice or pay attention to your own circumstances. Ask for understanding. Give the problem to your healing Guide and let it go.

The energy enters through your crown center, down to the base center, up and out your hands. Imagine the incoming energy as a shaft of light entering your crown chakra, filling the chakra pipeline, one then another, and breaking off to flow through your arms and legs. One woman with the gift of second sight sees the chakras like a cane beginning with the third eye and rising to the crown where it bends down like the cane's shaft to include the other chakras.

The purpose of a Reiki session is to balance the flow of energy through the chakras. The energy will adjust each chakra spin to allow appropriate energy flow to each of them. All you need to do is put your hands on or above each chakra and they will adjust themselves.

The energy you pick up through your palm chakras may feel like spirals, an electrical charge, or a pressure. Or you may not feel much at all at first. It is okay. Trust and keep stating your intentions. It is a practice, a learned process. The energy can do no harm. Use it, trust it enjoy it.

If, or when, you feel the need to move your hands, do so. The energy will ebb and flow as it is drawn to certain areas and then stops. When the flow stops then it is time to move your hands to the next chakra. Five to ten minutes above each chakra is enough. If you become over-whelmed, too hot, or begin feeling sick (taking on some of the symptoms of the client), lift your hands up and off.

There are many ways of clearing your hands. You can shake off the excess energy and let it drain into the earth. You can burn off the excess by moving your hands a safe distance above a candle flame. Some practitioners will keep a bowl of salt water nearby to dip their hands into. Washing them in a sink helps, but I like to limit this to the beginning and end of the session, so I do not have to leave the room and break the energy. Put your hands back down on the client when you are ready.

Taking on symptoms of the client is often a process in stimulating the energetic connection between client and practitioner. It creates some empathy and compassion. It is a way for you to understand where and why to move your hands. Remember: Reiki protects you, but to be safe, engage your mind and intention by stating the protection mantra, "Nothing but good comes from me and nothing but good comes to me."

You can also do some type of protective light work. Surround yourself with white light.

After her first attunement, at her first Reiki share, one woman wept with the emotions of each person who got on the table. She was forced to sit and meditate to connect with the group rather than put her hands down. She left weepy and exhausted. Try as she did, it was several shares before she learned why she was so eager to take on another person's issues. Her own lesson involved learning to love herself above all else. She learned to give the person energetic strength for their own healing and not to enable them by taking on their pain and sufferings and thus take away their personal lessons. She was in a word, enabling.

Reiki has a built-in preventative for any possibility of energy depletion in the practitioner. In channeling energy for another, the energy first revitalizes the practitioner. The healer receives a healing with each laying-on of hands. This two-fold advantage thus assures that the practitioner is built up, strong, filled up. What a beautiful message of giving and receiving!

The energy drawn by the recipient, however, is first utilized by the channel, the practitioner and thus is available for use with both parties. Therefore, when you do a Reiki session, you draw Reiki and are cleansed also. Double benefits!

Reiki is self-strength, and by keeping oneself strong, the energy that channels through during Reiki healings is, in turn, pure and strong.

As a new Reiki practitioner, it is important for you to be confident. Your confidence will build as you use your Reiki. Trust the forces working with you. Trust that your intentions to heal are creating a healing space and that healing is taking place whether you "see" it or not. Any emotional or spiritual issues that present themselves are gifts from the Higher Source to sort through and heal. My experience is that these issues are spotlighted for learning and examination. Your own study and meditation into personal issues and attitudes will encourage a deeper understanding of yourself and your relationship around the present moment. The here and now. Release, healing, enlightenment, and personal growth are the subject of hundreds of self-help books.

As a channel you will begin to feel lighter and more in control as you learn to understand energy and how you as a spiritual body can live in cooperation with the physical being.

A Reiki practitioner should cleanse their own energy paths and centers often by doing routine self-healings to keep their chakras open and their energy field free from "debris" which can be many things, from negative thoughts about self and others, to pain and trauma taken into the body from myriads of sources. Because the energy channeled through you as a practitioner will first heal the vessel, it becomes important to work on personal issues so that the energy moving through you to your clients will be stronger.

~ 14 ~
The Reiki balance

"Wherever two or more are gathered...."

With One Healer:

Because of the limitations of language, the exact title for an hour of receiving Reiki is difficult to give a name. The word "treatment" is colored by its widespread usage in the medical field. The word "session" has connotations of counseling. Reiki is both and more! The team healing comes with connotations of expectation. I like the term balance. It was coined by one of my students turned Master/Teacher. I like it because giving and receiving Reiki is balance, balance between the parties involved and balance within the spiritual, mental, and physical bodies. Feel free to choose a title you are comfortable with.

In a Reiki balance session, the practitioner will provide a safe, comfortable place. The room should have subdued lighting, perhaps soothing music playing for relaxation and to help buffer outside noise. A running fountain or a candle adds a nice soothing touch. It will become a space of healing and needs to reflect such.

The practitioner will ask the recipient to lie on their back and take several deep breaths, to relax. The practitioner will ask for the Reiki to flow, ask for protection and guidance and thank Spirit for assistance and the blessings of the present moment. He/she will start at the crown center at the top of the head and work down through the seven energy centers to the feet. Then the recipient will turn over and the chakras are worked down the back including the backs of the knees. The entire treatment takes an hour or so. The recipient will lie still, in a relaxed position. The practitioner will leave his/her hands on each energy center for 5-7 minutes. His/her hands will often feel warm, but not always. They may feel cold. The recipient may feel light tingling sensations, see colors, feel lighter, see light. Often there is a calm, peaceful feeling of relaxation. Often a client will fall asleep, which is fine.

Holding the hands out in the aura just above the body is sometimes more powerful than touching the person. You can feel the energy moving and feel the differences in blocked and releasing energy. Sometimes it will tingle or feel like throbbing points. Sometimes it will feel like rubbing the edge of a balloon.

Conversation during the treatment is possible but not encouraged as the whole purpose is to free the mind of the tangles and whirlwinds that sometimes one cannot seem to get free of.

Remember to keep yourself in a comfortable position so you do not get too tired or uncomfortable. If you are focusing on your leg going to sleep or your back in a crunch you are not available to concentrate on the energy flow.

During a session it is important to put your hands on each of the chakras and the feet because the purpose is to balance the chakras so they will run smooth, thus, the body is better able to heal itself. I also like to turn the client over and "work" the back chakras. If you are not in a place to have the client lie down, then have them sit and move your hands parallel with each other down the front and back while they sit in a chair. Parallel your hands down stopping at each chakra for the allotted time.

You will find many hand positions printed in different books. Use them as you choose but take to the Reiki table your own blessed

In Touch with Reiki I

intuition and move to places you feel guided to. Be discreet and respectful of the recipient and do not touch anywhere that could cause embarrassment or discomfort. Some people will react to the different positions. One woman was very uncomfortable with the heart position, and many are uncomfortable with the throat. Watch that your hands do not get too constricting, so they feel like choking. Often on the solar plexus, belly, and root your hands will be drawn to unusual angles, and positions. Follow your instincts while being aware of the recipient's needs.

One position used in difficult physical healings is to put hands one on top of each other, doubling the immediate intensity. I have done this myself and as a group with a pile of many hands in a situation on a difficult neck, or back, or with extreme pain.

Using both hands, shape a triangle above the pain point to create a focal point for healing energy to move through or to release. Often you will be able to see the energy inside the triangle your hands create. You may see a color or see it moving like strings or like heat rising off the asphalt.

When the hands-on portion of the Reiki session is over the practitioner will want to sweep the aura three times from head to toe. I like to sweep in a zig-zag method like sawing. This will disburse any released negativity and separate you from the client. The motion is a simple sweeping with the arms and hands toward a window or door. Another option is to sweep the energy down the body and into the earth for grounding. It is beneficial to ask the Spirit Guides to turn this energy into something positive. Visualize the particles becoming a rainbow or flower pedals.

Doubts about the validity of this portion of the session were put to rest after a Reiki share was held in my living room. My cat lay in the chair at the bottom of the table. He vomited all over the chair and floor during the night!

The next step, after sweeping, is to smooth the aura from feet to head. In a slow, deliberate motion move your hands up the body to raise the recipient's vibrational level and ground them. Palms down, hands together and move from the feet upwards. The client will feel the warmth.

Some people do a symbolic shining or circling three times of the recipient's halo to finish off the session.

Caution the recipient from getting up from the table too quickly. Encourage the recipient to take the session with them the rest of the day and try to return to it when outside interferences get too complicated and demanding. They may enjoy perhaps the best night's sleep they will have had in days. Months?

As a new Reiki practitioner and user, you will join the Drink Water police force! Remind your clients and yourself to drink water. Effects of a Reiki session will last for upwards of three days.

Share Reiki only if you have been invited to do so. You cannot force Reiki; the acceptance or rejection is up to the recipient not the practitioner. As a practitioner you are a channel not a director. If you are in a place where you believe the energy could be beneficial, but that the explanation will be awkward or too time consuming, ask the Angels/Spirit Guides of the person to accept the Reiki for them.

If a person has asked for healing and you do not feel like they are taking it, then know that your intentions to heal are just that and it is up to the recipient to accept and use the energy. You cannot direct or control the energy. You are the vessel, the conduit, the channel, not the director. Go back to your mantras for self-encouragement. Ask your healing guide for direction and guidance.

Do not direct the energy into a narrow focus because our view is very limited compared to the wisdom of Universal Life Force energy. If there are specific areas that you or the client want to address, ask for healing and ask that healing come to the area on all levels and for the highest good of all concerned. This broad, encompassing prayer covers a large area so the primary prayer concern expands healing by including any and all people, places and things associated with the issue. The prayer grows and magnifies and stretches to touch many.

For example, if you happen to be working with a bicycle injury and expand the prayer then the prayer can include the person whose car the bicyclist ran into!

Another example, a woman was on the table and had bitterly cold hands. She said her hands were always cold and her wrists always hurt. She raised her hand to look and said, "These are mother's hands."

I asked, stunned, "Whose?"

"My hands look just like my mother's." She went on to talk of the issues she had with her mother and realized she needed to reclaim her own hands. I like to say she re-membered the issues and the strength of her own hands.

Had we limited the work to the coldness of her hands and the pain in her wrists, the maternal, emotional issue would not have surfaced. We would have limited the scope of the healing and the physical symptoms would have had an unhealed, comfortable place to return.

I also believe the woman's mother received healing and every situation they had engaged in relating to this particular issue. The woman took responsibility for her hands and released her mother. This created a healing space, not a space for blame and hurt.

During a balance, specific areas may "call" to you through your intuitive feelings. Trust those gut feelings and work to develop them as they will direct you. To become more intuitive there are many, many books available.

There may be "hot" spots on the body. Your hands will be attracted to places where energy is stuck. When the block is removed your hands will cool down. When the energy flows smoothly there will be no hot spots or spots that will suck your hands in.

The highest benefits in a Reiki balance are attained by relaxing and enjoying the Reiki, trusting that the energy is working for the highest and best good, and allowing spiritual reconnection to work with its own knowledge and wisdom. Work within the security of well-being and contentedness by allowing the energy itself to work.

Concentrate on placing your hands above the seven major chakras, front and back, knees, feet, and palms of the hands. This coverage will guarantee a complete balance.

Remember that you are a channel, a vessel. You are not the healing energy.

I have seen Reiki work on all levels. I have seen physical symptoms intensified for quickened healing. I have seen physical symptoms, even intense pain, alleviated and I have seen physical symptoms bypassed and emotional issues surface. Several sessions (I recommend three very close together) and/or attunements are recommended for thick or complex issues because the negative energy can wrap itself around organs or hide or be so thick the body cannot process a complete release during one session. But do not doubt or dismiss the possibility of miracle healings.

Remember that the energy you are sending will work itself to every place it needs to be for the moment. If you sit at the crown chakra and channel healing for an hour the body will get appropriate healing! While the movements and procedures are designed to facilitate easy and quick healing and to assist the body, any hands down position will work. Stressing yourself over proper healing techniques hinders the flow of pure Spirit because your own fears will use the energy.

With more than one or a group of healers:

There are two lines of thought concerning the placing of many hands on one person. One theory is to join the intentions and then place hands all at once on the body. I think this is too strong a surge of energy if the person on the table is new to energy work. I think that practitioners should place their hands at intervals so the increased energy can flow more smoothly. I think the same for removing the hands, that they should not all be removed at the same time.

Working with others will decrease the amount of time on the body. A chakra balance/Reiki session lasts an hour or so. This type of healing should last 15-30 minutes, depending on the number of people involved.

Another caution involves a person who is new to energy. I would not work long on this person as the release may be unsettling. Be sure all who get up from the table are grounded.

Place people on each chakra, making sure each chakra is attended to. Watch for male and female root placements for the comfort of all involved. Also, keep people on either side of the client as balanced as possible.

One position used in group healing for when the recipient is on their back is to lay alternate hands down the spine like choking a baseball bat (the Louisville slugger position), from the throat to the root chakra. It creates a cocoon, an embryonic feeling of absolute warmth.

In Reiki shares one nice closing gesture is to have everyone hold hands making a circle for the healee to lie in. The energy of everyone involved is then focused on a swirling sphere. It is a real power surge. Those in the circle will feel an energy push when the recipient has had enough.

~ 15 ~
Using Reiki for distance healing

With the second level Reiki attunement, the student learns three of the Usui Reiki symbols. One is specifically for sending distance healing. But with this first attunement know that your prayers will be intensified so you may send the intention of Reiki along with your prayer concerns.

When sending energetic prayer, you need to give the intended healing somewhere to go if it is refused. If the person you are praying for does not accept the healing energy maybe their home or workplace will, or their plants will, or their animals will. The energy then acts as a space clearing, creating, perhaps a more peaceful atmosphere for the recipient's healing to occur.

Sometimes I ask that the next person who enters the room accept the energy. If the intended person is in the hospital, then this may be a nurse or a doctor or a family member who needs strength and knowledge.

If you are praying for a situation to be blessed, add "and all concerned" to the prayer. For example, if you are praying for a house to sell, pray for the right and perfect buyers and that all concerned with the transition be blessed. This includes then the realtor, the bankers, the moving company employees, the person who pumped the gasoline for the moving truck. The prayer is extended and as those people receive prayer blessings, they pass them on to those they touch. This way prayers cover an area beyond our knowledge and increase the blessings many times over. One woman on the prayer team who asked for prayer wrote back to say she saw the prayers as pink hearts traveling through space to her. A gentleman who was in a car wreck said he could feel the prayers of passersby as he was transported in the ambulance.

I have been a part of a prayer team on the internet for four years. The result of many sending prayer is miraculous and compassionate and comforting. We attempt to pray with no conditions, offering prayer for all the people concerned in a prayer request. We pray for the "bad" guys as well as the "good!"

One tough request concerned a young woman who was sexually abused. Requests involving violence and injustice create an opportunity to practice non-judgement. We are forced to choose what stand to take. Are we the judge and jury? Or are we aspiring to look without judgement at the soul of the person whose actions caused the pain and suffering? It does not mean we think sexual assault is okay, by any means. But it does mean we are forced to look at the perpetrator as a person, too. A rapist was an innocent child once. How does a person become violent? How does a person get to the point of addiction? What about the murderer, the car thief? I believe the perpetrators need our prayers as much or maybe even more. Is that a judgement? Humm. And I, too, struggle with that dilemma.

On the prayer team we are also asked to include "and all concerned" for those going into surgery or to a meeting or court hearing or starting a new job. As the prayers expand to all concerned, the possibilities are endless, and we are no longer in charge. The Creator is put in charge. Now that is a relief, to me!

Begin to leave Reiki in the chair you sit in at the movies or in church or on a pillow of one who is sick. Leave it on the wheelchair you push or the stroller or the grocery cart. A few minutes of Reiki is better than none for the next person who accepts it. Ask your guides to see that the energy is used to the best for all concerned. It is much like prayer; the intention of these energetic blessings is honored on a spiritual level.

Another way to spread healing and to help yourself is to bless your food. Bless what you drink. And bless everyone who has come into contact with what you eat and drink. Imagine this extended prayer as you bless the farmer, the truck driver, the marketing department, the cashier, the cook, and the waitress. All concerned.

And because food and water make a body run, eating becomes an act of reverence and responsibility. Everything you put into your body becomes a part of your field, of who you are, have been, and are creating. Make it easy for your physical body. Help your body to function to its fullest capability.

Ingest healthy, blessed nutrients. I do not propose food you do not like or purchased from the health food store. I believe that the body can deal with chips and chocolate (and fries!) as long as adequate nutrients are also taken in. I believe the body will begin to refuse those foods (and destructive behaviors) that are not for the highest good of the energies which compose your physical being.

~ 16 ~
Self-healing

...[W]e do not act in a void. Everything we do has an impact on everyone else. The thoughts and words that we bring into the world possess an energy that exists far beyond us.
Andrew, *Writing the Sacred Journey* 31

Peace on this planet begins with each individual walking here. It begins with you. Bring it to yourself and you bring it to others.

Perform Reiki in silence or in a meditative state whenever possible. When it is not possible use your Reiki anyhow. You do not always have to have a spiritual atmosphere to perform a spiritual act!

It is important to use your Reiki on yourself as often as possible. During clearing you will work on one chakra a day, up through all seven for three consecutive rotations. But after the initial period it is also important to do self-healings. You will want to be the clearest possible vessel for Reiki to pass through. If this is your intention then you will become a lighter and more peaceful and loving individual, affecting all people, places, and things around you.

Try to access as much Reiki as you can. Discover and drop your baggage. Let it surface and clear yourself. Do not be afraid of it. Forgive. Forgive yourself. Forgive others. Co-create your universe. Live how you wish to live. Do you choose peace? Joy? Love? Fear? Anger? Do you wish to give situations from your past control of your today? I know a divorced couple who hold so much anger towards each other it controls their relationship with their child.

Your attitudes and actions will change as you access Reiki. You will become more aware of the relationships between energy beings. We are all energy, so we are all one! And as you heal yourself others around you will relate to the new you. Many will be curious and want to learn what you have. You will be spreading healing on some level everywhere you go.

When your issues come up write them down and put the note between your hands and Reiki them. Issues will surface in layers. But remember, because one layer of a situation comes to you, and you work it out does not mean that issue is off the list! It may return several times before the root cause is discovered and dealt with.

If you are in pain or are trying to come to terms with a crisis or some buried problem, ask your Spirit guides to allow you to identify the root of the discomfort or perhaps ask for enlightenment through a dream. Ask that you be allowed to remember the dream and begin to work through the situation. Your guides will understand your discomfort and stay with you through the sorting out and dismantling process. (But they cannot interfere with your situation unless invited. It is called free will.) Reiki will reinforce you in any, and all, of these endeavors in that it gives you the strength of the Universal Life Force to cleanse and expand and enlighten. And what better support can you ask for?

Use Reiki to sleep. When doing your self-healings, place your hands upon the place you intuit as necessary and ask for healing. Instruct the Reiki when to stop its flow. Ask it to flow, say, for 60 minutes. This becomes an activity of complete trust.

If you have trouble sleeping, call the Reiki to you during the fitful times to help you relax. Surround yourself with white light and breathe it deep into your body. Hands on your belly or heart are quite relaxing. Image your favorite quiet place or draw in your imagination the perfect place of comfort and tranquility.

Go there with Reiki and sleep in the peace of wholeness. Join hands with your Spirit guides and feel their soothing presence.

There are chakra healing tapes/CDs you can buy to sleep with or do meditations with, the music changing every 5-7 minutes as you move through the chakras. Performing complete balances on yourself will grow your knowledge of the energy and your awareness of the different chakras and their relation to your overall health.

A practice that is beneficial for keeping your auric field cleansed is to "fluff" your aura. This is the process of combing through the auric field, waving your hands around you, like kneading it. The energy movement will keep your field free moving and eliminate places for negative things to "stick" and begin to create blocks. It also prevents your layers from falling in upon each other. This movement is beneficial if you have been in a large crowd, if you have been in a stressful situation, if you are feeling sluggish or are just down for no apparent reason. Like combing your hair, it makes you feel refreshed and lighter. And this in turn opens you to more energy and light so you step easier and closer to who you really are.

One way to test yourself to see if your chakras are open is to snap your fingers above the chakra. If the snap is dull, like a thud then the chakra is not functioning at its optimum level. An open chakra will be a sharp snap.

A position to boost energy is to place the right hand on the breastbone and the left on the belly. This is a tremendous 3:00pm position when the day has worn you down. It can be done for 5-7 minutes in your chair, in the comfort of a bathroom stall, or lying down.

~ 17 ~
The chakras

Each individual chakra is related to a particular organ, a particular emotion, color, and musical vibration. Without going into too much detail, note the following for details on the positions and a brief description of the focus of each. This very limited information was taken from notes in many texts. There are many, many good books written on chakras. Brief information is also given about them in most energy/healing related publications.

7TH CHAKRA – The crown – spirituality, transcendence

The crown is located at the top of the head, the "soft spot" location. This chakra is the site at which we connect to the universal energy. Spiritual love, at-one-ness with all that is, compassion, peaceful love towards all are qualities available at this chakra. Often, we perceive this energy as light and our connection to it as rays of light reaching from our crown to the universe and from the universe into our crown.

The physical and emotional dysfunctions centered here include sensitivity to pollutants, chronic exhaustion, epilepsy, Alzheimer's, depression, obsessional thinking, and confusion. Also, seizures, shock, paralysis, and stroke. This area will balance brain hemispheres. Come here for total integration of physical, mental, emotional, and spiritual bodies. Work in this area to find a sense of purpose and connection to the universe/Spirit.

In the front position work with the upper brain, motor cortex right eye, some sinuses and ear. The glands are the pineal and thalamus.

In the second or back position work with the occipital lobe, cerebellum, medulla oblongata, brainstem, and vision center. This includes the pituitary and the back of the third eye chakra.

This back position encompasses the third eye also. Work here for balance, to eliminate dizziness and to correct high or low blood pressure. Work here for concerns with alertness, mood swings and manic-depressive traits. Work here for dream recall and when searching for a sense of purpose.

The color is violet (or violet-white). The element is light. Its musical vibration is B. The crystals and minerals are amethyst, diamond, and alexandrite.

Self-Healing:
Just above the ears place the palms of your hands on each side of your head. Your fingertips should touch on the crown of your head.

Healing others:
Touch the heels of the palms together at the top of the head with the fingers coming down to just behind the base of the skull.

6TH CHAKRA – The third eye, the brow - wisdom, intuition

The third eye is located in the center of the forehead between the two eyes. It is the intuitive energy center, the center that sees the larger picture. Visions, intuitive abilities, and symbols are all operations associated with the third eye. Ones who are gifted with intuitive abilities, through any sense, will be interested in keeping this chakra open and smooth flowing.

Areas governed here include the lower brain, left eye, ears, nose, and nervous system. The glands are the pituitary, thyroid and parathyroid. This is the area for the tonsils, vocal cords, trachea, and pharynx. Here metabolism is regulated.

Here also find an element of communication which is related to a sense of belonging and one's sense of self-worth. Here is how our speech and thought patterns relate to what we think of who we really are. The degree of intuitive connection and understanding will affect our outlook and thus our everyday expressions.

Dysfunctions include problems with headaches, poor vision, neurological disturbances, glaucoma, nightmares, learning difficulties, and hallucinations. It also includes throat problems and flu, tonsillitis, and speech problems. Blood pressure, lymphatic drainage, stroke, and nervous problems can be treated here. It is also connected to self-esteem and how we speak about who we are and what we want and believe. In my experience many men have trouble keeping their third eye chakra open.

The color is indigo (a dark purple blue). The element is light. Its musical vibration is A. The crystals and minerals are Lapis Lazuli, purple fluorite, and clear quartz.

Self-healing:
Front position: Place the palms on the forehead.
Back position: Cup or cradle the base of the skull with your palms. Fingers can point to the neck. Light pressure on the base of the skull will work several acupressure points.

Healing others:
Let your palm rest on the lower part of the head with your fingers at the base of the skull. Pressure can be placed with the fingertips. Another position is to put your hands, with palms together, like in prayer. Place your hands parallel with the spine, fingers pointing towards the feet. Let the client's head rest with the base of their skull sitting on the

first knuckle of the thumb. Align your fingers straight down each side of the spine until the energy is smooth running down both hands.

Holding front and back of this chakra at the same time (on yourself or others) is a good position for creating balance.

5TH CHAKRA – The throat – communication, self- expression

The throat chakra is concerned with the expression of the self through the voice and the mind. It deals with communication of feelings and thoughts. Any form of creativity that involves language, is connected with this chakra. Speaking up, releasing emotion, and breathing (essential to the Life-Force) are focused here. In my experience women have trouble keeping their throat chakra open.

The bronchial and vocal apparatus, the lungs and the alimentary canal are the physical areas governed in the throat chakra. The gland is the thyroid.

Dysfunctions include problems with sore throats, neck ache, thyroid problems, tinnitus, asthma, perfectionism, inability to express emotions, and blocked creativity. Here is where we block what we desire. Here is where fear of failure is addressed.

The color is blue. The element is ether. Its musical vibration is G. The crystals and minerals are turquoise and aquamarine.

Self-healing:
Front: With the heels of your palms together, wrap your hands, fingers pointing back, around your throat. Point your fingers up to the base of your skull.

Back: You can also hold your hands on your collar bones fingers pointing down the back.

Healing others:
Front: Wrap your hands around the client's throat with fingers meeting above the Adams apple. Keep them loose.

CAUTION: Some people are very sensitive to this position. Be sure your hands are not so close as to give the client a sense of choking.

Back: Lay hands together with the fingers of one hand touching the heel of the other across the collar bone.

Working on the shoulders releases the "shoulds." Shoulds are what we take into our belief system from another's belief system. What that person thinks we should be doing, thinking, or wearing. Whatever others have told us we should or should not be doing. It is society telling us how to parent, what we should drive, what we should eat, what our body should look like. Releasing the shoulds releases burdens of another's mandates. It also releases our own false mandates as directed from the ego self or the self who has bought into the beliefs of another. It is releasing all that is not about being true to our authentic selves.

4TH CHAKRA - The heart - love, compassion

The heart is the seat of harmony, trust, love, gentleness with self and others. It deals with attachment and detachment, with the need to feel secure, validated and loved. The emotional components of self-esteem are located at this chakra. This chakra is also associated with healing, both of the self and of others. Here is your capacity to love, your sensitivity to loving others unconditionally. Here is seeing the soul self of others, not the physical self. Here is openness to life and all the situations life offers.

The heart chakra is also the point at which the higher energies of the head and spirit meet the lower energies of the material body. As such it is a central point of balance within the connection of mind, spirit, and body. Heart, of course, but also blood, and the vagus nerve, along with the circulatory system, are governed in this area. Lungs are also included in this chakra. The gland is the thymus.

Related to this chakra are high blood pressure, heart disease, cancer, co-dependency, melancholia, and fears of betrayal. Also centered here are roots of allergies, immune system disorders, and infections. All lung and respiratory problems are centered here. Emotional elements of this area are jealousy, anger, and hate.

The color is green or pink. The element is air. Its musical vibration is F. The crystals and minerals are emerald, tourmaline, jade, and rose quartz.

Self-healing:
Front: Hands just above breasts, the fingers touching other at center of the sternum.

Back: Hands on the ribs, fingers pointing towards the spine. There are chakras in the nipples so be sure that they are open. Open them by rotating your hands, palm above the nipple, and pulling up and out.

Healing others:
Front: Hands just above the breasts the fingers of one hand touching the heel of the palm of the other. Or make a T-formation with your hands with one hand in the very center of the body, between the breasts, one hand parallel with the collar bone.

CAUTION: Be very aware of where your hands are. If you have any indication that the client is uncomfortable with your hand placement hold them above the body 6-8 inches.
Respect the client's privacy and their body at all times.

3RD CHAKRA - The solar plexus - personal power

The solar plexus is the location of the power of the self. It is the residence of the ego and is concerned with categorizing, separating, and planning. It is the seat of mental energy and creativity. When this chakra is in balance the body is centered, the power of the self is linked to the soul and earth mission. This chakra is all about self-will, respect for self and others. Not being in balance here can lead to giving up personal power, can create a determination to control others, and manifest problems with perfectionism.

The stomach, liver, gall bladder, pancreas, and nervous system are the physical areas governed here. Dysfunctions include stomach ulcers, digestive problems, chronic fatigue, allergies, diabetes, cirrhosis, over sensitivity to criticism, and the need to be in control. Here is fear also and paranoia.

The color is yellow. The element is fire. The musical vibration is E. The crystals and minerals are yellow topaz, citrine, amber and tiger's eye.

Self-healing:
Front: Hands just under the breasts a few inches above the navel. Touch fingers at sternum.
Back: Hands over same position on the back.

Healing others:
Front: Hands just under the breasts a few inches above the navel. Touch fingers of one hand to heel of palm of the other at the sternum.
Back: Same position on the back. The belly may start to rumble when the energy starts flowing well!

2ND CHAKRA – The spleen, belly - emotional balance, sexuality

This chakra is located 2-3 inches below the navel. It is associated with relationships with other people, emotional needs, and boundaries (including sexual issues), intimacy, beginnings, and endings. The reproductive system is the area of the body governed. The glands are the gonads. This is the chakra of forming relationships, or desire and sexuality. It is about giving and receiving pleasure on all levels, spiritual, mental, and physical.

Problems associated with this area are impotence, frigidity, bladder and prostate dysfunction, lower back pain, unbalanced sex drive, emotional instability, and feelings of isolation. It is also the area of diabetes. It, with the solar plexus, has to do with symptoms of cirrhosis, infections, and digestion issues. It also is associated with feelings of acceptance.

The color is orange. The element is water. The musical vibration is D. The crystals and minerals are coral, moonstone, and fire opal.

Self-healing:
Front: Hands below the belly button a couple of inches meeting at fingertips.
Back: Hands just below waist, fingers meeting at spine or pointing down.

Healing others:
Same positions.

1ST CHAKRA - the root, the base - survival and safety

The root chakra is located at the base of the spine, the coccyx. It is associated with the physical body. Any issue that involves survival and/or manifesting what is necessary for life on the physical plane is affiliated with the root chakra. Issues of safety and security also arise in the root chakra, as does our sense of physical boundaries. It is about grounding and staying in the physicalness of this existence. We are spiritual bodies having a physical experience and so it is important to remain grounded in all that we do and realize the effect our existence has on this earth plane.

The areas of the body governed are the spinal column and kidneys. The glands are the adrenals. It also affects parts of the reproductive system, as well as the bladder and parts of the digestive system.

Dysfunctions include osteoarthritis, mental lethargy, spaciness, and incapacity to attain inner stillness. Work here for reproductive problems, constipation, diarrhea, bladder problems, suicidal tendencies, and frequent illnesses.

The color is red. The element is earth. Musical vibration C. Crystals and minerals are ruby, pyrite, garnet, and hematite.

Self-healing:
Front: Hands over lower abdomen. If you can, put your hands on your "bottom."
Back: Sit on your hands!

Healing others:
Front: Just above pubis, fingers touching in the center of the body. Keep your hands above the client 6-8 inches.

CAUTION: Because of the sensitivity of this area be VERY aware of where your hands are at all times. You have no reason to touch another's sexual places during a Reiki balance. If you are uncomfortable with this position, or suspect that the client is, place a hand on each side of the hips, holding the pelvic area in healing. This will send energy across the body and through the area.

Back: Hands just above the tail bone, fingers meeting at the spine.

~ Chapter 18 ~
Additional positions utilizing one or more chakra

FOR BACK PAIN:
Hold one hand at the neck and the other at the tail bone to hold the spine in healing energy. This is good for any back problems and to help the client stand straight and courageous in their mission.

FOR SCIATICA:
On either side of the body hold the hip and the foot chakra allowing energy to run down the leg. One hand will pull, and one will push the energy.

FOR RELEASING TOXINS:
Hold one hand under the client on the pelvic bone and place one hand above the client on the side of the belly to hold the adrenals in healing. The position is just below the belt line. Place your fingertips at the spine and the other hand just above it. Hold this position for 5-10 minutes or longer. If you get too "hot" or overwhelmed just remove your hands.

FOR BALANCING HEAD AND HEART:
Place one hand an inch or so above the heart and the other 6-8 inches above the crown chakra. Hold until you can feel the energetic connection. Move the hand above the crown down while moving the hand above the heart up. Like a push-me pull-you! The energy should move at an equal flow up and out, forcing the other to move up or out at the same rate and distance. This is a good position if the person is going to be making decisions that involve head and heart.

Susan Rea Caldwell

~ Reading list ~

There are many wonderful Reiki books available. And many more on healing and self-development. I encourage you to seek Spiritual connection through the written word. Reading helps you to connect with others' experiences and thoughts. Remain free to accept or reject any thought that does not resonate with the truth you feel in your soul. Rejecting often solidifies your own beliefs. Explaining yourself helps solidify your truths and so you are free to grow and explore and expand.

For information on energy healing, two great books are Jack Angelo's Hands on Healing: A Practical Guide to Channeling your Healing Energies and Michael Bradford's The Healing Energy of Your Hands. They describe the energy field of the body, how the energy flows and works. They also have some excellent exercises, meditations, and visuals for learning to feel and work with the energy.

The Diane Stein Essential Reiki is the handbook. I refer to her book often. She includes an excellent bibliography for Reiki and hands on healing.

One Degree Beyond is Janeanne Narrin's text on how to incorporate Reiki into your everyday life and use it in making decisions and healing emotional baggage. Her recapitulation of the history of Reiki and the homage she pays to Dr. Usui give us an interesting look into the reality of what his process was in bringing the Reiki healing system to us.

Karyn Mitchell has written an excellent and informative book, Reiki: A Torch in Daylight.

Bodo J Baginski and Shalila Sharamon co-authored a fine book, Reiki Universal Life Energy. This book details a history of the Reiki Master lineage through Hawayo Takata.

Frank Arjava Petter writes Reiki Fire: New Information about the Origins of the Reiki Power: A Complete Manual from a fascinating Master's perspective, and The Original Reiki Handbook of Dr. Mikao Usui which delves into Dr. Usui's original text on the hand positions and healing formats.

Paula Horan has written several books on creating personal change through the evocation of Reiki energy. Empowerment Through Reiki: The Path to Personal and Global Transformation is one of them. She describes the history of Reiki before Petter's discoveries. Abundance through Reiki is another text excellent for using Reiki in all areas of your life.

There are several styles of Reiki. What I teach is Traditional Usui. Some groups offer further attunements and continuing degrees. One is Sai Baba Reiki of which I am trained. One is Karuna Reiki which I have studied.

The International Center for Reiki Training, (www.reiki.org) has a newsletter and has recently introduced a new version of Reiki called Reiki Fire. The web is full of Reiki information and practitioners offering free distance healings, chat room opportunities, and information.

For spiritual growth I found many of my personal truths in the following:

First and foremost: The Conversations with God series, by Neale Donald Walsch. It has been the greatest eyeopener I have ever experienced on my journey. The text gives me hope and confirms my innermost beliefs. It is the most comprehensive and loving text I have ever read on the how and why of life!

The Course in Miracles was my lifesaver and guide when I received my attunements, but the Conversations series was much easier for me to understand. Marianne Williamson is a student and excellent teacher of The Course in Miracles and brings that often difficult text into more understandable and usable theories. She has a website and lecture series: Marianne.com.

The Game of Life and How to Play It, by Florence Scovel Shin, was written in the 1920s but is still excellent in suggesting ways of attaining enlightenment and understanding and how to co-create a positive universe for ourselves. It is here I learned of the Divine Plan.

During that same period, Catherine Ponder was writing excellent books on prosperity and healing. Any of her books are recommended. Healing Through the Ages, the Dynamic Laws of Healing, and Open your Mind to Prosperity is also helpful.

Gary Zukav's Seat of the Soul describes the concept of this life being a school and how to "play" in it.

Go to the bookstore and browse through the self-healing and/or new age books. Pick them up and feel the energy.

~ Bibliography ~

A Course in Miracles. Foundation for Inner Peace, 1992.

The American Heritage College Dictionary. 3rd Edition. Boston: Houghton, Mifflin Co, 1993.

Andrew, Elizabeth. *Writing the Sacred Journey: The Art and Practice of Spiritual Memoir.* Skinner House Books. Boston, MA, 2005.

Angelo, Jack. *Hands on Healing*. Rochester, VT: Healing Arts Press, 1994.

Baginski, Bodo J and Shalila Sharamon. *Reiki Universal Life Energy*. Mendocino, CA, Life Rhythm, 1988.

Bourbeau, Lise. *Listen to Your Body*. Saint-Sauveur des Monts (Quebec), Editions E.T.C. Inc, 1989.

Bourbeau, Lise. *Heal Your Wounds and Find Your True Self.* Saint-Sauveur des Monts (Quebec), Editions E.T.C. Inc, 2001.

Bourbeau, Lise. *Your Body's Telling You: Love Yourself!* Saint-Sauveur des Monts (Quebec), Editions E.T.C. Inc, 2001.

Bradford, Michael. *The Healing Energy of Your Hands*. Freedom, CA, The Crossings Press, 1993.

Burnham, Sophy. *The Ecstatic Journey*. New York, NY: Ballantine Books, 1977.

Carter, Karen Rauch. *Move Your Stuff, Change Your Life*. New York, NY: Fireside, 2000.

Emerson, Barbara. *Self-Healing Reiki*. Berkeley, CA: Frog, LTD, 2001.

Esquivel, Laura. *Like Water for Chocolate*. New York, NY: Random House. 1992

Fuentes, Star. *Light Language - Beginner's Manual*. 1992.

Garfield, Charles, Cindy Spring and Sedonia Cahill, *Wisdom Circles*. New York, NY, Hyperion, 1998.

Hay, Louise L. *Heal Your Body*. Carson, CA., The Hay House.

Herman, Deborah Levine with Cynthia Black. *Spiritual Writing*. Hillsboro, OR, Beyond Words Publishing, Inc., 2002.

Horan, Paula. *Empowerment through Reiki*. Twin Lakes, WI, Lotus Light-Shangri-La, 1996.

Horan, Paula. *Abundance through Reiki*. Twin Lakes, WI, Lotus Light-Shangri-La, 1995.

International Association of Reiki Professionals, www.iarp.org.

The "I AM" Discourses. St Germain Foundation, Schamburg, IL, St Germain Press, 1996.

Mitchell, Karyn. *Reiki: A Torch in Daylight*. St. Charles, IL, Mind River Publications, 1994.

Motz, Julie. *Hands of Life*. New York, NY: Bantam Books. 1998.

Narrin, Janeanne. *One Degree Beyond*. Seattle, WA, Little White Buffalo Publishing Cottage, 1998.

NumberQuest - http://numberquest.com/numbers.html

Petter, Frank Arjava. *Reiki Fire*. Twin Lakes, WI, Lotus Light Shangri-La, 1997.

Petter, Frank Arjava. *The Original Reiki Handbook of Dr. Mikao Usui*. Twin Lakes, WI: Lotus Light Shangri-La, 1999.

Ponder, Catherine. *Open Your Mind to Prosperity*. Marina del Rey, CA, DeVorss and Co., 1971.

Ponder, Catherine. *The Dynamic Laws of Healing*. Marina del Rey, CA, DeVorss and Company, 1966.

Rand, William. Reiki - *The Healing Touch. First and Second Degree Manual*. Southfield, MI, Vision Publications. 1998.

Redfield, James. *Celestine Prophecy*. New York, NY, Warner Books, Inc., 1997.

Ruiz, Don Miguel. *The Four Agreements*. San Rafael, CA, AmberAllenPublishing, 1997.
http://www.miguelruiz.com/agreements.html

Sai Baba Workshop booklet.

Shin, Florence Shovel. *The Game of Life and How to Play It*. Marina del Rey, CA, DeVorss, 1925.

Stein, Diane. *Essential Reiki*. 4th printing. Freedom, CA, The Crossings Press, 1996.

Suess, Dr. *Green Eggs and Ham*. New York, NY, Random House, 1988.

Thayer, Steven and Linda Sue Nathanson, *Interview with an Angel*. Gillette, NJ, Edin Books, 1997.

Twyman, James. E-site James@emissaryoflight.com

Unity Publications. *Daily Word*. Unity Worldwide Ministries, Unity Village, MO,

Walsch, Neale Donald, *Conversations with God. Book 1*. Charlottesville, VA, Hampton Roads, 1996.

Walsch, Neale Donald, *Conversations with God. Book 2*. Charlottesville, VA, Hampton Roads, 1997.

Walsch, Neale Donald, *Conversations with God. Book 3*. Charlottesville, VA, Hampton Roads, 1998.

Walsch, Neale Donald, *Friendship with God*. New York, NY, G. P. Putman's Sons, 1999.

Williamson, Marianne. *A Return to Love*. New York, NY, HarperPerennial, 1992.

Zukav, Gary. *Seat of the Soul*. New York, NY, Fireside, Simon and Schuster, 1998.

~ About the author ~

Susan Rea Caldwell, MA, RM, wears many hats. She received her BA from the University of Kentucky in 1994 and in 1996 her MA from Marshall University in English and Creative Writing.

As a writer she has received several grants from the Kentucky Foundation for Women, has published many short stories and two novels, Betty Rea and Joseph's Journey, a collection of vignettes, Tales from smack in the middle of New Hampshire Drive and a few miles beyond: The Gordon and Ivan series.

She has practiced energy balance therapy since 1996 when becoming a Usui Reiki Master/Teacher. She has written manuals for each level of Reiki training, In Touch with Reiki - Manuals for Teachers and Students Levels I, II, III.

Susan is an Akashic Records consultant, guiding a client through a dialogue with the keepers of the events of their soul's personal journey.

As a labyrinth facilitator, certified through Veriditas@ she leads labyrinth walks for personal healing, for global healing, for guidance and direction, and for expanding creativity.

As a workshop leader she facilitates Julia Cameron's Artist's Way providing intense and gratifying path for seekers on their path to personal truth. She also hosts play shops in making prayer flags and vision boards.

As an artist, Susan creates fabric collage wall hangings using repurposed and vintage items, particularly hand-crafted items.

Susan Rea Caldwell

In Touch with Reiki I

Susan Rea Caldwell

www.ingramcontent.com/pod-product-compliance
Lightning Source LLC
Chambersburg PA
CBHW070324190526
45169CB00005B/1738